NCWC'S NUTRITION 101 WORKBOOK

A. Sehatti, RN, MSN
Family Nurse Practitioner

NCWC/Amend-Health Press

ISBN 978-0-578-87863-8 (paperback)

Weight Management	Weight Loss	High Cholesterol	Diabetes
Healthy Eating	Nutrition		

Includes biographical references

Printed and bounded in the United States of America
First Printing: March 2021
Revised May 2021, April 2023

Published by:
NCWC/Amend-Health Press
AKA Nutritional Counseling and Weight Control Clinic
51 E. Campbell Avenue, Suite 129 - 154
Campbell, CA 95008
United States
www.NCWC-AmendHealthPress.com
www.EatActThinkHealthy.com

About the Author

A. Sehatti is a registered nurse and family nurse practitioner. She received her bachelor's degree in nursing from University of Pennsylvania and her master's degree in nursing from University of California, Los Angeles. Aside from her clinical work at such places as Caltech Health Center, UCLA, and Stanford Medical Center, she has over forty years of experience in educating adults and children on weight management, nutrition, and total wellness. A. Sehatti is highly dedicated to making a difference in people's lives. She currently works as a nutritional consultant and health educator at a private practice that she established in 2005 in Northern California. It has been the reward of witnessing people reach their health and wellness goals that has inspired the author to write books and share the tools that have helped her clients with her readers.

Books Published by A. Sehatti

BUILDING A STRONG SENSE OF SELF
Embarking on the Journey of Change
The Inner Control Is the True Control - Book 1

ACCOUNTABILITY AND EMPOWERMENT
A Four-Step Strategy for Overcoming Resentment
The Inner Control Is the True Control - Book 2

THE INNER CONTROL IS THE TRUE CONTROL
WORKBOOK, SECOND EDITION
Inspirational Scripts

A TOOL FOR LETTING GO OF RESENTMENT AND ANGER
Short. Straightforward. Transformative.

A WORKBOOK FOR OVERCOMING RESENTMENT
Mindfulness Scripts

A HANDBOOK FOR DEALING WITH SUGAR
CRAVINGS AND DEPENDENCY
NCWC's Nutrition 101 Series

21-DAY LOG BOOK FOR ACHIEVING WELLNESS GOALS
NCWC's Nutrition 101 Series

Ncwc's Nutrition 101 Workbook is a collection of nutrition education handouts and note-taking worksheets.

Please be informed that this workbook is *only* designed as such to enhance your learning experiences when you are having tele-health or in-person nutritional consultations.

Ncwc's Nutrition 101 Workbook is organized according to the nutrition education curriculum offered by A. Sehatti, RN, MSN, FNP at NCWC (Nutritional Counseling and Weight Control Clinic).

To attain greater outcomes in achieving health goals, it is strongly recommended that one uses this workbook in conjunction with the *21-Day Log Book for Achieving Wellness Goals*.

Please note that the knowledge shared in this book can change over time based on the latest scientific findings that are discovered.

Moreover, the information provided by the author is not intended to be complete or exhaustive nor is it a substitute for the advice and/or prescription offered to you by your primary care provider.

Contents

CHAPTER 5

CHAPTER 6

1

Weight Control

MAINTAINING WEIGHT
Total calories burned = Total Calories taken in
per day   Per day

LOSING WEIGHT
Total calories burned > Total Calories taken in
per day   Per day

GAINING WEIGHT
Total calories burned < Total Calories taken in
per day   Per day

Questions	Yes	No
Should I follow the celebrity endorsed diets?	☐	☐
Will skipping breakfast suppress my appetite and help me lose weight?	☐	☐
Will eating one meal a day help me lose faster?	☐	☐
Is rapid weight loss okay?	☐	☐
Should I go on "a diet" to lose weight?	☐	☐
Should I avoid carbs to lose weight?	☐	☐
Will drinking 12 cups of water a day help me lose weight faster?	☐	☐
Should I drink protein shakes after workouts?	☐	☐
Is running better than walking for exercise?	☐	☐
Is it all about how much calories I take in and burn out?	☐	☐

Factors Affecting the Amount of Calories You Burn in a Day

◇ Resting Metabolic Rate
◇ Physical Activity
◇ Thermogenic Effect of Food

1. RESTING METABOLIC RATE

_____
_____
_____
_____

a. Heredity

_____
_____

b. Body size: surface and composition

_____
_____
_____
_____
_____
_____
_____

c. Age and Sex

_____

_____

_____

_____

_____

d. Hormones

_____

_____

_____

_____

_____

_____

_____

e. Temperature / Environment

_____

_____

f. Dieting

_____

_____

_____

_____

2. PHYSICAL ACTIVITY

3. THERMOGENIC EFFECT OF FOOD

Factors Affecting the Amount of Calories You Take in a Day

◇ Neurotransmitters
◇ Gut Peptides
◇ Hormones
◇ Habits and Psychosocial Factors
◇ Environment (i.e., Friends)
◇ Others (i.e., Culture and Finances)

1. NEUROTRANSMITTERS

_____
_____
_____
_____
_____
_____
_____
_____
_____
_____
_____
_____
_____
_____
_____

2. GUT PEPTIDES

_____

_____

_____

3. HORMONES

_____

_____

_____

_____

4. HABITS AND PSYCHOSOCIAL FACTORS

_____

_____

_____

5. ENVIRONMENT (i.e., FRIENDS)

_____

_____

_____

_____

6. OTHERS (i.e., CULTURE AND FINANCES)

_____

_____

_____

2

Proteins

- Meat (E.g., Chicken, Turkey, Fish)
- Meat Substitutes:
  - Egg
  - Legumes
  - Legume-Derived Foods (E.g., Tofu)
  - Nuts
  - Yogurt
  - Milk
  - Cheese

1 gram of protein = 4 calories

PROTEINS

Essential   Non-essential
Amino acids   Amino acids

COMPLETE PROTEINS

MEAT AND MEAT SUBSTITUTES

VERY LEAN 0-1 GRAM FAT	LEAN 3 GRAMS FAT	MODERATE-HIGH 5 OR MORE GRAMS FAT	HIGH-FAT 8 OR MORE GRAMS FAT
Poultry: Chicken or turkey white meat with no skin 1 oz	Poultry: Chicken or turkey dark meat with no skin 1 oz	Poultry: Chicken or turkey ground or dark meat with skin 1 oz	Pork: Spareribs, ground, or sausage 1 oz
Fish: Fresh or frozen cod, flounder, halibut, trout, lox 1 oz	Salmon or herring 1 oz	Any fried fish 1 oz	Peanut butter *(unsaturated fat)* 1 TBSP
Egg whites 2	Beef: USDA select or choice lean trimmed of fat 1 oz	Beef: Most products, meatloaf, corned beef 1 oz	Processed Luncheon meats *(with 8 grams of fat per ounce)* 1 oz
Egg substitues, plain 1/4 cup	Pork: Lean (i.e., fresh, canned, cured, or boiled ham; tenderloin; center-loin chop) 1 oz	Pork: Top lion, chop, Boston butt, or cutlet 1 oz	Bacon 3 Slices (20 slices/lb)
Legumes: (i.e., Cooked beans or lentils) *(carbohydrate exchange)* 1/2 cup	Lamb: Roast, chop, or leg Veal: Lean chop, or roast 1 oz	Lamb: Rib roast, ground Veal: Cutlet (ground/cubed) 1 oz	Hot Dog 1
Fat-Free/Low-Fat cottage cheese 1/4 cup	4.5%-Fat cottage cheese 1/4 cup	Ricotta cheese 1/4 cup	Cheese: All regular cheeses 1 oz

MEAT AND MEAT SUBSTITUTES (Cont'd)		
VERY LEAN **0-1** **GRAM FAT**	**LEAN** **3** **GRAMS FAT**	**MODERATE-HIGH** **5 OR MORE** **GRAMS FAT**
Cheese with one gram fat or less 1 oz	Grated Parmesan cheese 2 TBSP / 1 oz	Feta or Mozzarella cheese: 1 oz
Shellfish: clams, crab, lobster, scallops, shrimps 1 oz	Oysters 6 Medium	Egg *(High in cholesterol)* 1
*Seitan *(Carbohydrate exchange)* 1 oz	***Tempeh *(Carbohydrate exchange)* 1 oz	Bacon 2 Slices
**Tofu *(Carbohydrate exchange)* 1 oz		**Tofu *(Carbohydrate exchange)* 4 oz

Adapted from Exchange Lists for Meal Planning - ADA

*Seitan (hydrated gluten/wheat gluten): 1 oz contains 105 calories, 0.5 gram of total fat (0.1 gram of saturated fat), 21 grams of protein (carbohydrate exchange)

**Tofu (soy product): 1 oz contains 21 calories, 1 gram of total fat (0.2 grams of saturated fat), 2 grams of protein (carbohydrate exchange)

***Tempeh (soy product): 1 oz contains 55 calories, 3 grams of total fat (0.6 grams of saturated fat), 5 grams of protein (carbohydrate exchange)

Your Individual Plan for Meeting
Your Daily Protein Requirement

MEAL	MEAT OR MEAT SUBSTITUTES (COMPLETE PROTEINS)	PORTION SIZE
BREAKFAST		
LUNCH		
DINNER		

_____

_____

_____

_____

_____

3

Carbohydrates

- Grains (E.g., Bread, Cereal, Rice, Pasta)
- Vegetables
- Fruits
- Legumes (E.g., Beans, Lentils, Peas)
- Dairy (E.g., Milk, Yogurt, Cheese, Ice Cream)

1 gram of carbohydrate = 4 calories

Claims	True	False
Carbohydrates are fattening.	☐	☐
Carbohydrates are the dietary culprit behind obesity.	☐	☐
Bread and pasta are fattening.	☐	☐
A carbohydrate-restricted diet helps me lose weight faster.	☐	☐
A low-carbohydrate, high-protein diet is good for me.	☐	☐
Sugar makes children hyperactive.	☐	☐
Brown sugar is more nutritious than white sugar.	☐	☐
I should consume artificial sweeteners and other sugar substitutes instead of raw sugar.	☐	☐
Sugar causes diabetes.	☐	☐
Refined Carbohydrates make me fat.	☐	☐
I should take fiber supplements to make sure that I'm getting enough fiber.	☐	☐

CARBOHYDRATES

```
                    CARBOHYDRATES
                    ↙          ↘
               Simple          Complex
              ↙   ↓   ↘         ↙    ↘
                              Starch  Fiber
                                       ↙   ↘
   Glucose  Fructose  Galactose
                                    Soluble   Insoluble
```

_____

_____

_____

_____

_____

_____

_____

_____

_____

_____

_____

_____

_____

_____

_____

_____

_____

_____

_____

Simple Carbohydrates

» Ingredient labeling is required on all foods that have more than one ingredient. Read these listings carefully.

» A food may be high in added sugar when any form of sugar appears in the first 3 or 4 ingredients.

» A food may also be high in added sugar when several of any form of sugar appear in its ingredients.

» The followings are used in ingredient listings to describe sweeteners that are added:

◇ Sucrose
◇ Fructose
◇ Maltose
◇ Lactose
◇ Glucose
◇ Dextrose
◇ Honey
◇ Molasses
◇ Brown sugar
◇ Barbados sugar
◇ Beet sugar
◇ Syrup
◇ Brown rice syrup
◇ Malt syrup
◇ Maple syrup
◇ High-fructose corn syrup
◇ Corn syrup
◇ Barley malt syrup
◇ Buttered syrup
◇ Corn sweetener
◇ Fruit juice concentrate
◇ Agave nectar
◇ Evaporated cane juice
◇ Cane juice
◇ Barley malt
◇ Ethyl Maltol

Read the ingredient listings carefully. Eating these sugars may cause stomach discomfort, bloating, gas, and loose stools (they may pass unabsorbed into the colon).

◇ Large amounts of *lactose* (especially in people who are lactose intolerant)

◇ Large amounts of *fructose*.

◇ Large amounts of *sucrose*.

◇ *Stachyose*. Used commercially as a bulk sweetener. Natural ingredient in green beans, soybeans, and other beans.

◇ *Raffinose*. Used as the base for Sucralose (*Splenda*-artificial sweeteners). Natural ingredient in beans, cabbage, brussels sprouts, broccoli, asparagus, and whole grains.

◇ Small amounts of *sorbitol, mannitol, xylitol, lactitol, maltitol* (alcohol sugars).

◇ Small amounts of *lactulose*. A synthetic sugar.

◇ *Olestra* (olean, sucrose polyester). Fake fat: in some potato chips, granola bars, crackers, salty snacks

◇ *Lignin*. A dietary fiber.

◇ *Inulin* (fructan). A dietary fiber. Added to some yogurts.

Complex Carbohydrates

_____
_____
_____
_____
_____
_____
_____
_____
_____
_____
_____
_____
_____
_____
_____

ENDOSPERM

SHELL
(BRAN)

GERM

GRAIN SEED

Adapted from: The Whole Grains Council

Consuming whole grains in recommended amounts can help reduce abdominal fat (waist-to-hip ratios) and the risk of:

◇ Heart disease and stroke: lowers cholesterol levels

◇ Cancer: Cancers of digestive system (GI cancer) and hormone-related (breast and prostate cancers)

◇ Diabetes (Type II)

Foods that list the following whole-grain ingredients as the first one on their label's ingredient list are whole grain.

- ✓ Brown rice
- ✓ Wild rice
- ✓ Bulgur
- ✓ Graham flour
- ✓ Oatmeal
- ✓ Whole grain corn
- ✓ Whole oats
- ✓ Whole rye
- ✓ Whole wheat

Foods with the following labels or ingredients are usually *not* whole-grain products:

- ◇ Multi-grain
- ◇ Stone-ground
- ◇ 100% wheat
- ◇ Cracked wheat
- ◇ Seven-grain
- ◇ Bran

The color of the food (i.e., bread) does not mean that it is whole grain.

Whole Grain Foods and Flours

The followings are some examples of generally accepted whole grain foods and flours when they include the bran, germ and endosperm:

◇ *Barley*: Look for whole barley, hulled barley, or hull-less barley. The fiber in barley lowers blood cholesterol levels.

◇ *Bulgur*: FDA has defined all bulgur as whole grain. It has more fiber than such foods as quinoa, oats, millet, corn, or buckwheat. It cooks rapidly.

◇ *Corn* (includes whole cornmeal and popcorn): It contains a high level of antioxidants. Look for the word "whole corn." Avoid when the label says, "degerminated."

◇ *Millet*: On an ingredient list, it is most likely whole millet.

◇ *Oats* (include oatmeal): When they are in the ingredient listings as "oats," "oatmeal," or "oat groats," they are most likely whole oats. Research Studies have shown that oats, like barley, contain a special kind of fiber that help lower blood cholesterol level. They also protect blood vessels against LDL cholesterol because they contain a unique antioxidant.

◇ *Rice*: Brown rice as well as black or red rice are whole grains. It is easily digested; Therefore, it may be ideal for a restricted diet (i.e., gluten-free diet).

◇ *Rye*: A "rye bread" label doesn't mean that it is whole grain. Look for such words as "whole rye" or "rye berries" in the ingredient listings. The fiber in rye may rapidly help you feel full.

◇ *Whole Sorghum* (milo): It is a gluten-free whole grain and therefore it can be an option for a gluten-free diet.

◇ *Teff*: It has more iron and calcium than many other grains.

◇ *Triticale*: It is a hybrid of wheat and rye.

◇ *Wheat* (includes spelt, emmer, durum; it can also include such forms as bulgur, cracked wheat or wheat berries): Look for "whole wheat" as the first ingredient. Plain "wheat" legally means that it is refined wheat.

◇ *Wild rice*: It is most likely whole wild rice when it is in the ingredient listings.

Oilseeds and such legumes as flax, chia, sunflower seeds, soy, or chickpeas are not considered whole grains by the WGC, the AACC International, or the FDA.

Source: The Whole Grains Council

Pseudo Grains

Pseudo-grains are included since their nutritional values and cooking preparation are very similar to whole grains:

◇ *Whole Amaranth*: Contains a high level of an amino acid (lysine) that may be negligible or not be in many grains.

◇ *Buckwheat*: It is most likely whole buckwheat when it is in the ingredient listings. It has high levels of rutin (an antioxidant that may prevent cholesterol from building up in blood vessels).

◇ *Quinoa*: It is high in proteins — complete protein.

Source: The Whole Grains Council

Soluble and Insoluble Fiber

FIBER CONTENT OF FOODS

FOOD	AMOUNT	FIBER (g)	CALORIES
Cooked black beans	1 cup	15	227
Cooked pinto beans	1 cup	15.4	245
Cooked garbanzo beans (chickpeas)	1 cup	12.5	269
Cooked lentils	1 cup	15.6	230
Fresh raw strawberries	1 cup	3	48
Fresh raw blueberries	1 cup	3.6	86
Fresh apple with the skin (e.g. red delicious)	1 medium	4.9	125
Fresh orange	1 large	4.4	87
Fresh kiwi	1	3	64
Fresh fruit juice	1/2 up	0	Variable
Fresh cucumbers, with peel	1/2 cup slices	0.3	8
Raw broccoli	1 cup chopped	2.4	31
Raw carrots	1 cup	3.4	49
Cooked asparagus	1/2 cup	1.8	20
Raw avocado	1/2 (75 g)	5	120
Raw bell pepper	1 cup	1.8	46
Raw lettuce (e.g., iceberg)	1 cup chopped	0.7	8
Fresh vegetable juice	1/2 cup	0	Variable
Raw almonds, unroasted	1 oz (~ 23 whole)	3.5	164
Raw walnut halves	1 oz (~14 halves)	1.9	185

Source: USDA and Healthline

Serving Sizes

FRUITS	
60 Calories **12 grams of Carbohydrate**	
Fresh apple 1 small	Watermelon 1 cup
Fresh orange 1 small	Fresh mango 1/2 small
Fresh kiwi 1	Banana 1 small
Fresh grapefruit 1/2 large	Fresh grapes 1/2 cup
Fresh nectarine 1 small	Fresh pineapple 3/4 cup
Fresh blueberries 3/4 cup	Cantaloupe 1/3 small
Fresh strawberries 1 1/4 cup	Fresh unsweetened fruit juice 1/2 cup
Fresh plums 2 small	Dried apricots 8 halves
Fresh tangerines 2 small	Dried figs 2 Medium

Adapted from Exchange Lists for Meal Planning - ADA

VEGETABLES

**25 Calories
5 grams of Carbohydrate**

Raw vegetables: Broccoli Carrots Celery Bell Pepper Cucumber 1 cup	Cooked vegetables: Beets Asparagus Carrots Brussels sprouts Cabbage Cauliflower 1/2 cup

Adapted from Exchange Lists for Meal Planning - ADA

STARCHY VEGETABLES AND LEGUMES

**80 Calories
15 grams of Carbohydrate
0-1 gram of Fat**

Corn on cob 1/2 cob	Sweet potato/Yam 1/2 cup
Mashed potato 1/2 cup	Boiled potato 1/2 cup or 1/2 medium
Baked potato with skin 1/4 large	Cooked beans, lentils, peas 1/2 cup

Adapted from Exchange Lists for Meal Planning - ADA

GRAINS

80 Calories
15 grams of Carbohydrate
0-1 gram of Fat

Bread 1 slice	Cooked rice 1/3 cup
Bagel 1/4 or 4 oz	Cooked pasta 1/3 cup
English muffin 1/2	Corn/Flour tortilla (6") 1
Granola (low-fat) 1/4 cup	Cooked cereal 1/2 cup
Bran cereal 1/2 cup	Graham cracker (2 1/2" square) 3
4" Pancake (1/4 in. thick) 1	Waffle (4 1/2 in. square) 1
Biscuit (2 1/2 in. across) 1	Pita (6 in. across) 1/2
Popcorn (no fat added) 3 cup	Pretzels 3/4 oz

Adapted from Exchange Lists for Meal Planning - ADA

DAIRY		
12 grams of Carbohydrate **8 grams of Fat**		
NON-FAT **0-3 GRAMS FAT** **90 CALORIES**	**LOW-FAT** **5 GRAMS FAT** **120 CALORIES**	**WHOLE** **8 GRAMS FAT** **150 CALORIES**
Skim or 1% milk 1 cup (8 oz)	2% Milk 1 cup (8 oz)	Whole milk 1 cup (8 oz) Evaporated whole milk 1/2 cup (4 oz)
Non-fat or low-fat soy milk 1 cup (8 oz)	Soy milk 1 cup (8 oz)	Kefir 1 cup (8 oz)
Plain nonfat yogurt 1 cup (8 oz)	Plain low-fat yogurt 1 cup (8 oz)	Plain whole milk yogurt 1 cup (8 oz)
Fat-free cottage cheese 1/4 cup	Skim or part-skim milk cheeses such as: Ricotta 1/4 cup Mozzarella 1 oz	Any regular cheese (i.e., American, Monterey, Swiss, or cheddar) 1 oz

Adapted from Exchange Lists for Meal Planning - ADA

SUMMARY	
Fruit	12 grams of carbohydrate 60 Calories
Vegetables	5 grams of carbohydrate 25 Calories
Starchy Vegetables and Legumes	15 grams of carbohydrate 80 Calories
Grains	15 grams of carbohydrate 80 Calories
Dairy	12 grams of carbohydrate 90-120 Calories

Adapted from Exchange Lists for Meal Planning - ADA

1 gram of carbohydrate = 4 calories
1 gram of fiber = 0 calories
1 gram of sugar alcohol = 7 calories

Your Individual Plan for Meeting
Your Daily Carbohydrate Requirement

GRAINS AND STARCHY VEGETABLES (INCLUDING LEGUMES)	15 grams of carbohydrate 80 Calories	_____ Servings per day
FRUITS	12 grams of carbohydrate 60 Calories	_____ Servings per day
VEGETABLES	5 grams of carbohydrate 25 Calories	_____ Servings per day
DAIRY	12 grams of carbohydrate 90-120 Calories	_____ Servings per day

MEALS	GRAINS, STARCHY VEGGIES, or LEGUMES	VEGTABLES	FRUIT	DAIRY
BREAKFAST				
MID AM SNACK				
LUNCH				
MID PM SNACK				
DINNER				

4

Fats

Oils
Avocados
Nuts
Cream Cheese
Peanut Butter
Butter
Sour Cream
Cream
Seeds
Lard
Coconut
Bacon
Salad Dressing
Mayonnaise
Olives

1 gram of fat = 9 calories

```
                            FATS
                      ↙      ↓      ↘
            Fatty Acids  Triglycerides  Cholesterol
              ↙     ↘                  ↙      ↘
        Saturated   Unsaturated      HDL      LDL
                      ↙     ↘
                   Mono      Poly
```

A. TRIGLYCERIDES

_____

_____

_____

_____

_____

_____

_____

_____

_____

_____

_____

_____

_____

_____

_____

B. CHOLESTEROL: HDL AND LDL

C. FATTY ACIDS: UNSATURATED

» MONOUNSATURATED FATTY ACIDS

» POLYUNSATURATED FATTY ACIDS

» TRANS FAT

D. FATTY ACIDS: SATURATED

FATTY ACIDS		
5 grams of Fat **45 Calories**		
Monounsaturated	**Polyunsaturated**	**Saturated**
Olive, canola, or peanut oil 1/2 TBSP	Corn, sunflower, soybean, sesame, or safflower oil 1 tsp	Palm oil 1 tsp
Avocado 2 TBSP or 1/8 medium	Pumpkin or sunflower seeds 1 TBSP	Cream cheese 1 TBSP
Almonds or Cashews 6 nuts	Walnuts 4 halves	Coconut 2 TBSP
Peanuts 10	Coconut (shredded) 2 TBSP	Bacon 1 slice
Pistachios 12	Margarine stick or tub 1 tsp	Butter stick 1 tsp
Pecans 2	Mayonnaise 1 tsp	Lard 1 tsp
Olives (small) 10	Salad dressing (regular, all varieties) 1 TBSP	Sour cream 2 TBSP
Olives (large) 5	Salad dressing (regular, mayonnaise-type) 2 tsp	Cream or half & half 2 TBSP

Adapted from Exchange Lists for Meal Planning - ADA

Your Individual Plan for Meeting Your Daily Fat Requirement

Total calories per day: _____

Total fat per day: _____ grams

Total saturated fat per day: _____ grams

Examples of Healthy Dietary Fats
(Monounsaturated Fatty Acids):
Nuts, Avocado, Extra Virgin Olive Oil
(Caution: Portion Size Matters!)

_____
_____
_____
_____
_____
_____
_____
_____
_____
_____
_____
_____
_____
_____

5

The Disease Triangle

The disease triangle is a conceptual model that may show the relationship among the environment, host, and pathogen.

This model is based on the fact that even if a species is highly susceptible, not all individuals within the community would have the same level of susceptibility.

◇ *Agent*: The pathogen (infectious or non-infectious) causing the disease
◇ *Host*: An individual may have genes that protects it against the disease (resistance)
◇ *Environment*: The right environment makes an individual vulnerable to the disease (i.e., weak immune system caused by poor diet, stress, lack of exercise, and inadequate sleep)

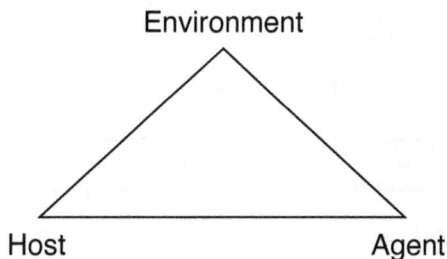

Environment

Host   Agent

Carcinogenesis

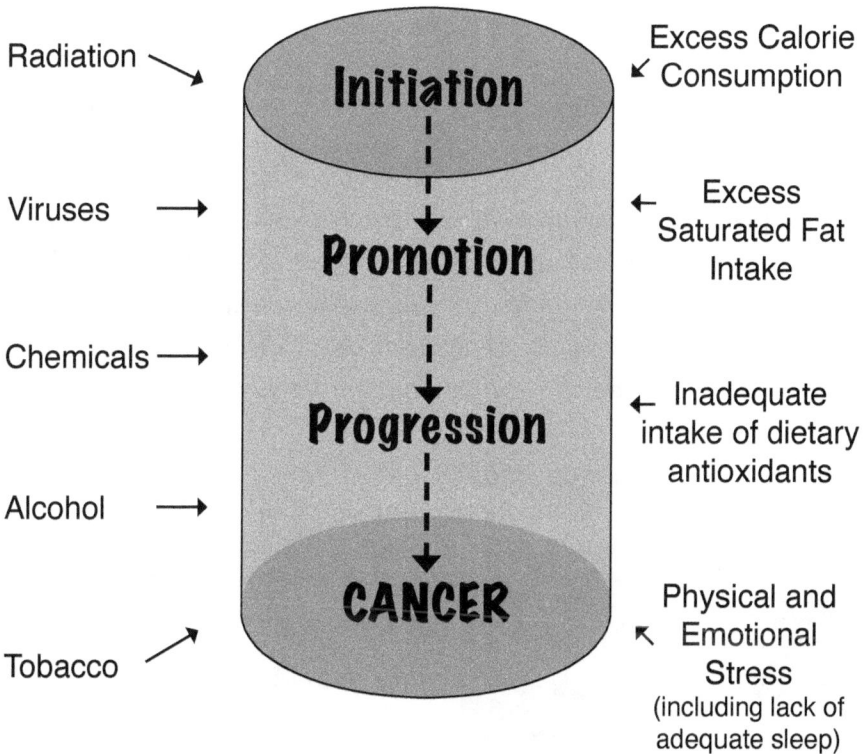

Radiation →

Viruses →

Chemicals →

Alcohol →

Tobacco →

Initiation

Promotion

Progression

CANCER

Excess Calorie Consumption

Excess Saturated Fat Intake

Inadequate intake of dietary antioxidants

Physical and Emotional Stress (including lack of adequate sleep)

Adapted from NCBI (National Center for Biotechnology Information)

"Only 5–10% of all cancer cases can be attributed to genetic defects, whereas the remaining 90–95% have their roots in the environment and lifestyle.

The lifestyle factors include cigarette smoking, diet (fried foods, red meat), alcohol, sun exposure, environmental pollutants, infections, stress, obesity, and physical inactivity.

The evidence indicates that of all cancer-related deaths, almost 25–30% are due to tobacco, as many as 30–35% are linked to diet, about 15–20% are due to infections, and the remaining percentage are due to other factors like radiation, stress, physical activity, environmental pollutants , etc.

Therefore, cancer prevention requires: smoking cessation, increased ingestion of fruits and vegetables, moderate use of alcohol, caloric restriction, exercise, avoidance of direct exposure to sunlight, minimal meat consumption, use of whole grains, use of vaccinations, and regular check-ups."

Source: NCBI (National Center for
Biotechnology Information)

LIFESTYLE CHANGES FOR PREVENTION OF CANCER

◇ Be lean but not underweight.
◇ Be physically active and fit.
◇ Avoid/limit sugary food and drinks.
◇ Avoid/limit energy-dense foods.
◇ Eat vegetables, fruits, whole grains and legumes (include Variety).
◇ Avoid/limit of red meats (i.e., beef, pork and lamb).
◇ Avoid processed meats.
◇ Best to avoid but if consumed, limit alcoholic beverages to 2 for men and 1 for women per day.
◇ Avoid/limit eating salty foods.
◇ Avoids/limit foods processed with sodium.
◇ Avoid unproven supplements to protect against cancer.
◇ Do not use tobacco in any form.

Source: American Institute for Cancer Research

The Stress Response

AUTONOMIC NERVOUS SYSTEM

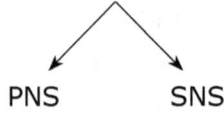

PNS   SNS

A. PARASYMPATHETIC NERVOUS SYSTEM (PNS)

_____

_____

_____

_____

_____

_____

_____

B. SYMPATHETIC NERVOUS SYSTEM (SNS)

_____

_____

_____

_____

_____

_____

_____

_____

Over-Stimulation of Sympathetic Nervous System

◇ Prolonged Elevation of Cortisol
◇ Loss of Cortisol Circadian Rhythm (i.e., Inversion of Rise-and-Fall of Cortisol Secretion)
◇ Eicosanoids Imbalance
◇ Others

1. PROLONGED ELEVATION OF CORTISOL

_____
_____
_____
_____
_____
_____
_____
_____
_____
_____
_____
_____
_____
_____
_____

2. LOSS OF CORTISOL CIRCADIAN RHYTHM

_____

_____

_____

_____

_____

_____

3. EICOSANOIDS IMBALANCE

_____

_____

_____

_____

_____

_____

_____

4. OTHERS

_____

_____

_____

_____

_____

_____

Chronic stress leads to prolonged elevation of cortisol levels in our blood. A high level of cortisol over the long term can lead to such health problems as the followings:

◇ Heart disease
◇ High blood pressure
◇ Digestive disorders
◇ Higher blood sugar levels
◇ Weakened immune system
◇ Auto-immune disorders
◇ Psychosomatic symptoms such as dizziness, muscle aches, or backaches
◇ Mental health problems such as depression and/or anxiety
◇ Premature aging

Stress Management

Gain insight and become aware.

BRAIN

System Measures to Boost
Your Immune System

Some Rich Sources of Fat Soluble Vitamins

Vitamin A
Red, orange and yellow fruits and vegetables and leafy greens:
◇ Carrots
◇ Cantaloupe
◇ Apricots
◇ Kale
◇ Spinach
◇ Broccoli
◇ Winter squash
◇ Red bell peppers
◇ Collards
◇ Turnip greens
◇ Baked sweet potato

Vitamin D
◇ Fortified milk
◇ Sun

Vitamin E
◇ Vegetable oils
◇ Wheat germ
◇ Whole-grain products
◇ Seeds
◇ Nuts and peanut butter
◇ Avocados

Vitamin K
◇ Green leafy vegetables such as: kale, spinach, turnip greens, collards, Swiss chard, mustard greens, parsley, and lettuce
◇ Vegetables such as Brussels sprouts, broccoli, cauliflower, and cabbage

Some Rich Sources of Water Soluble Vitamins

Vitamin C

Many fruits and vegetables such as: citrus fruits, watermelon, cantaloupes, strawberries, kiwifruit, red bell pepper, tomatoes, and broccoli

Vitamin B Complex

» **Thiamin (B1)**
◇ Green peas
◇ Whole-grain
◇ Enriched-grain products including bread, rice, pasta, tortillas and fortified cereals

» **Riboflavin (B2)**
◇ Milk and dairy foods
◇ Enriched bread and other grain products
◇ Lean meats
◇ Eggs
◇ Leafy green vegetables such as spinach

» **Niacin (B3)**
◇ High-protein foods including peanut butter, poultry, fish
◇ Avocado
◇ Enriched and fortified grain products

» **Vitamin B6 (Pyridoxine)**
◇ Baked potato
◇ Banana
◇ Fortified cereals
◇ Nuts
◇ Beans
◇ Chicken and fish

» **Vitamin B12**
  ◊ Milk and dairy foods
  ◊ Meat
  ◊ Fish (especially salmon)
  ◊ Poultry
  ◊ Eggs

» **Folate**
  ◊ Orange juice
  ◊ Spinach
  ◊ Romaine lettuce
  ◊ Broccoli
  ◊ Peanuts
  ◊ Avocado
  ◊ Enriched grain products and fortified breakfast cereals

_____

_____

_____

_____

_____

_____

_____

_____

_____

_____

_____

_____

6

Your Individual Plan for Meeting Your Wellness Goals

◊ Total calories per day: _____
◊ Total protein per day: _____ grams
◊ Total carbohydrates per day: _____ grams
◊ Total fat per day: _____ grams
◊ Total saturated fat per day: _____ grams
◊ Total cholesterol per day: _____ milligrams
◊ Total sodium per day: _____ milligrams

_____

_____

_____

_____

_____

_____

_____

_____

Daily Dietary Planning

The goal is to
stabilize blood sugar.

1. Avoid hunger
2. Eat 3 well-balanced meals at regular hours (sitting down and chewing well)
3. Eat complete proteins and whole grains at each meals
4. Eat healthy mid-morning and mid-afternoon snacks
5. Include selections from all food groups
6. Limit or avoid foods high in sugar, fats, and salt (i.e., fried foods, fast foods, pastry, soda, juice, jam, chocolate, chips, pickles, canned foods, etc.)
7. Do not eat for at least 2 hours before going to bed
8. Eat most of your calories before the evening
9. Drink 6-8 glasses of water daily

_____

_____

_____

_____

_____

_____

_____

_____

_____

DAILY GOAL		
FOOD GROUP	**CALORIES PER ONE SERVING**	**# OF SERVINGS RECOMMENDED**
GRAIN	80 calories	
STARCHY VEGETABLE AND LEGUME	80 calories	
VEGETABLE: RAW AND COOKED	25 calories	
FRUIT	60 calories	
DAIRY	90-150 calories	
MEAT AND MEAT SUBSTITUTE	35-100 calories	
FAT	45 calories	
SWEET AND ALCOHOL	Varying calories	

_____

_____

_____

_____

_____

_____

_____

_____

_____

_____

_____

_____

_____

_____

_____

_____

_____

_____

_____

_____

_____

_____

_____

_____

_____

_____

_____

_____

DAILY DIET

FOOD GROUPS	NUMBER OF SERVINGS				
	Breakfast	Snack	Lunch	Snack	Dinner
Grains					
Starchy Vegetables and Legumes					
Vegetables: Raw and Cooked					
Fruits					
Dairy					
Meats and Meat substitutes					
Fats					

Breakfast
One-hour time range: _____

Mid-Morning Snack
One-hour time range: _____

Fruit (one serving) + Dairy (one serving) (i.e., 1 fresh apple with the skin + 6 oz plain Greek yogurt)
Fresh fruit (one serving) + Nut (one serving) (i.e., 1 fresh orange + 1/4 cup unsalted almonds)
Raw veggies (1-2 serving) + Nut (one servings) (i.e., 1 cup raw baby carrots + 1/4 cup unsalted almonds)
Raw veggies (1-2 serving) + Dairy (one servings) (i.e., 1 cup raw baby carrots + 6 oz plain Greek yogurt)
Fresh fruit (one serving) + Raw veggies (one servings) (i.e., 1 fresh orange + 1 small raw bell pepper)

Lunch
One-hour time range: _____

_____

_____

_____

_____

_____

_____

_____

_____

Mid-Afternoon Snack
One-hour time range: _____

Fruit (one serving) + Dairy (one serving) (i.e., 1 fresh apple with the skin + 6 oz plain Greek yogurt)
Fresh fruit (one serving) + Nut (one serving) (i.e., 1 fresh orange + 1/4 cup unsalted almonds)
Raw veggies (1-2 serving) + Nut (one servings) (i.e., 1 cup raw baby carrots + 1/4 cup unsalted almonds)
Raw veggies (1-2 serving) + Dairy (one servings) (i.e., 1 cup raw baby carrots + 6 oz plain Greek yogurt)
Fresh fruit (one serving) + Raw veggies (one servings) (i.e., 1 fresh orange + 1 small raw bell pepper)

Dinner
One-hour time range: _____

_____

_____

_____

_____

_____

_____

_____

_____

_____

After Dinner

_____

_____

_____

_____

_____

_____

_____

_____

_____

Daily Activity Planning

The importance of physical activity in achieving and maintaining total wellness cannot be overemphasized.

Moving Around / Engaging in Light-Intensity Activities:

Definition: Any activity that we engage in, which increases the body's energy expenditure above the resting level.

Examples: Activities of daily living (i.e., self-care); cooking; washing dishes; watering the plants; taking out the trash; shopping; strolling around; walking the dog; yoga

Benefits: Staying active throughout the day helps us sleep better. It prevents weight gain; improves stomach motility and gastric emptying; lowers our blood pressure; reduces anxiety and helps prevent depression. These are just some of the benefits that accumulated activity throughout the day may offer us.

Engaging in Daily Aerobic Exercises / Cardio Workouts (Cardiovascular conditioning):

Definition: Any moderate-paced activity, sustained for at least 10 minutes, that increases our breathing and heart rate through continuous, repetitive, and rhythmic movement of the large muscle groups of arms and legs may be considered as an aerobic exercise.

Examples: Brisk walking, swimming, dancing, and jogging

Benefits: Among many other benefits, aerobic exercises deliver oxygen and nutrients to our tissues; improve our cognitive functioning; keep our blood vessel flexible and consequently improve our circulation, blood pressure, and cardiovascular health; stabilize our blood sugar levels; boost our immune system; reduce fatigue; lessen anxiety; and, improve our mood.

30-45 minutes of aerobic activities, 5-7 days per week, help us lose weight and maintain our weight loss; boost HDL (the good cholesterol) and consequently lower our risk of stroke, heart attack, or other cardiovascular diseases; stabilize our blood sugar and consequently help prevent type 2 diabetes or other endocrine problems such as PCOS (polycystic ovary syndrome); and, reduce the risk of developing colon cancer or other chronic health diseases.

Performing Muscle Strengthening Activities (2-3 times/week):

Definition: Any activity in which the repeated contractions of the major muscle groups (i.e., our abdomen, arms, legs, and chest) against a weight or force (i.e., our own body weight, free weights, weight machines, or exercise bands) are sustained for about 10 seconds or more may be considered as a muscle strengthening activity. (Lower intensity/higher repetition is recommended.)

Examples: Push-ups and sit-ups; pilates; yoga workouts; lifting weights; working out using dumbbells, bands, or weight machines

Benefits: One or more sets of 12 repetitions of such exercises performed two to three times per week improves our balance and helps prevent falls; strengthens our bones, reduces the rate of bone loss, and helps prevent osteoporosis; boosts our metabolism and helps us lose weight; and, improves our flexibility and endurance.

Performing Daily Stretching Activities:

Definition: Any activity in which we flex or stretch a specific muscle group while moving the related joint through its full range of motion may be defined as a stretching routine.

Examples: Yoga, neck rolls, standing hip rotations, etc.

Benefits: Stretching a few minutes per day improves our posture, flexibility, and range of motion; decreases muscle tension and helps prevent tension headaches, neck or back pain.

Limiting/Avoiding Sedentary Activities:

Definition: Sedentary activity may be defined as any activity that we engage in for an average of 8 hours or more per day, which doesn't increase the body's energy expenditure much above the resting level.

Examples: Lying down; sitting; watching TV; working/reading/ playing on a computer or cell phone; playing video games

Benefits: Limiting or avoiding sedentary activities is vital in maintaining our physical and mental health. Inactivity increases the risk of embolism (blood clots); stiffens our blood vessels and increases the risk of developing high blood pressure or other cardiovascular diseases; leads to weight gain and puts us at risk for type 2 diabetes, colon cancer, depression, and other health problems. In short, a sedentary lifestyle raises the risk of early morbidity and mortality.

Set a goal; commit to your goal by making realistic and achievable plans; and, be active while having fun;

Track your daily steps;

Set limits for such sedentary activities

as watching TV or playing electronic games;

Set reminders (i.e., on your phone) to take
short breaks for getting up and moving around
when you have to sit at a desk.

To turn your physical activity into a daily routine,
keep a daily log and aim for progression, not perfection
(overcome all-or-nothing way of thinking).

_____

_____

_____

_____

_____

_____

_____

_____

_____

_____

Please consult your healthcare professional before starting a new exercise program or workout routine, especially if you are diagnosed with such chronic health problems as hypertension, heart disease, diabetes, cancer, or arthritis.

Behavioral Changes:
Mindfulness

Gain knowledge, become mindful, take baby steps,
and gradually change your eating habits.

_____

_____

_____

_____

_____

_____

_____

_____

_____

_____

_____

_____

_____

_____

_____

_____

_____

_____

_____

_____

_____

Resources:

◇ *The Inner Control Is the True Control Workbook: Inspirational Scripts. 2nd Edition*

◇ *BUILDING A STRONG SENSE OF SELF: Embarking on the Journey of Change. (The Inner Control Is the True Control - Book 1)*

◇ *Accountability and Empowerment: A Four-Step Strategy for Overcoming Resentment (The Inner Control Is the True Control - Book 2)*

◇ *A Tool for Letting Go of Resentment and Anger: Short. Straightforward. Transformative.*

◇ *A Workbook for Overcoming Resentment: Mindfulness Scripts*

Supermarket Shopping: Food Labels

A. FOOD LABELS

» **Nutrition Fact**

1. Trans Fat
2. Serving Sizes
3. Calories
4. Saturated Fat*
5. Cholesterol*
6. Total Fat*
7. Sodium*
8. Total Carbohydrate
9. Added Sugar

*Use the Daily Value Rule

» **Ingredient List**

◇ _____
◇ _____
◇ _____
◇ _____
◇ _____
◇ _____
◇ _____

B. OTHERS

_____

_____

_____

_____

_____

Nutrition Facts

2 servings per container

2 | **Serving size**   **1 piece (88 g)**

Amount per serving

3 | **Calories**   **330**

% Daily Value*

6 **Total Fat** 16 g	**21%**
4 Saturated Fat 16 g	**31%**
1 *Trans* Fat 0 g	
5 **Cholesterol** 85 mg	**29%**
7 **Sodium** 410 mg	**18%**
8 **Total Carbohydrate** 41 g	**15%**
Dietary Fiber 0 g	**3%**
Total Sugars 22 g	
9 Includes 22 g Added Sugars	**43%**
Protein 8 g	**16%**

Vitamin D 0.4mcg 2% * Calcium 30mg 2%

Iron 1.8 mg 10% * Potassium 200 mg 4%

*The % Daily Value (DV) tells you how much a nutrient in a serving of food contributes to a daily diet. 2,000 calories a day is used for general nutrition advice.

Eating Out

General Tips

◇ Before going to unfamiliar restaurants, check the menu and find out nutritional information.

◇ Avoid hunger (i.e., don't skip meals before going out to eat).

◇ Try not to finish all the food on your plate because you don't wish to waste money or food. Ask to have half of your entree or dish to be bagged to go before starting to eat or ask for a box to do it yourself.

◇ Ask that salad dressing, gravy, sauces, mayo, sour cream, and guacamole to be served on the side. Request lemon wedges. Squeezing fresh lemon juice may help you to use less of the dressing, gravy, or sauce. Avoid croutons.

◇ Watch your portion sizes and choose water as a drink.

Breakfast/Brunch

◇ Breakfast sandwiches are usually high in calories, saturated fat, cholesterol, and sodium—especially, those on croissants or biscuits.

◇ Breakfast muffins (without butter or any spread) may have 340 to 630 calories and 2 to 8 grams of saturated fat. Doughnuts have 2-5 grams of saturated fat and 2-5 grams of trans fat. So, avoid these foods or limit the portion sizes.

◇ Be mindful of coffee drinks. Besides extra calories and sugar, they may add more saturated fat to your meal (Ask for non-or low-fat milk instead).

◇ Go for à La carte instead of buffet style when possible.

Lunch

◇ Sandwiches on whole wheat bread usually may be the best choices.

◇ Chicken, turkey, and lower-fat cheese (Swiss) are good choices for fillings. Mayo-laden salad-type fillings (i.e., tuna, chicken, etc.) are high in total and saturated fat. (Limit or avoid processed or luncheon meats.)

◇ Ask for one-fourth of an avocado instead of Mayo, Pesto, or other dressings.

Dinner

◇ Order salad as an appetizer (or part of the appetizer) to avoid eating bread; Some appetizers can be filling and replace a meal.

◇ Limit or avoid soups. They are high in sodium. Cream soups are high in total fat and saturated fat.

◇ Avoid dishes that are fried, made with cheese or cheese sauces, seasoned with fat, or have added gravies and creamy sauces.

◇ Avoid or limit red meat. Choose dishes with lean meats, fish, and poultry that are baked, broiled, boiled, or grilled. Better choices for red meat may be lean roast beef, roast veal, small lean steak (tenderloin or filet mignon), veal chop or pork chop cutlet. Remove the fat and skin as much as possible.

◇ Request veggies that are steamed, grilled, or roasted that are not prepared with sauce, butter, or margarine.

Desserts

◇ Share or eat smaller portions of your favorite high-calorie or high-fat desserts.

◇ Use Carbohydrate and Fat Exchange List in order to ensure balance.

◇ Sorbet or fresh fruits are great alternatives to ice-cream.

Others

_____

_____

_____

_____

_____

_____

_____

_____

_____

_____

_____

_____

_____

_____

HEALTHY EATING AT SOCIAL GATHERINGS

_____

_____

_____

_____

_____

_____

_____

_____

_____

_____

_____

_____

_____

_____

_____

_____

_____

_____

_____

_____

Tips for Making Better Choices During Holidays

Goal: Prevent weight gain.

Making small steps toward maintaining your weight during the holidays matters; it all adds up.
Practice moderation, not deprivation (portion control); be physically active; and, have pleasant holidays!

1. If you are celebrating with your family:
   ◇ Have a meeting and discuss your holiday eating/activity plans with them.
   ◇ Before parties or celebrations, come to an agreement with your children about such issues as drinking too much soda or eating too much sweets/candy.
   ◇ Go to the supermarket together as a family.

2. Make a grocery list on a full stomach and go to the supermarket with a full stomach.

3. Make better choices: It is much easier to pile up on calories when you have calorie-dense foods or drinks (i.e., foods or drinks that are high in calories and low in nutrients, such as baked goods, candies, salad dressings, sugary drinks, and soda).

4. It might not be a good idea to go to a party hungry—we are more likely to overeat when we are hungry.

5. Avoid drinking too much alcohol, which can weaken your resolve and lead to overeating—in particular, if you're drinking on an empty stomach.

6. Limit drinking sugary drinks (i.e., juice, soda, or coffee/tea drinks), which make it easy to quickly add a lot of calories to your diet.

7. Choose water as the beverage of your choice.

8. Go easy on dips, chips, salad dressings, sauces, and gravies, which can add a lot of calories and fat (in particular, saturated fat) to your diet.

9. Concentrate on healthy and natural foods that contain fiber, such as fresh veggies. Such healthy selections will:
   ◇ Suppress your appetite;
   ◇ Curb your cravings; and,
   ◇ Boost your metabolism (induced thermogenesis).

10. When you are serving yourself at a buffet:
    ◇ It may be a better choice to choose a few of your favorite hors d'oeuvres rather than a pile of everything that is offered.
    ◇ Take sensible portions so that you could avoid going back for seconds.
    ◇ Be mindful of walking around the buffet table or sampling from passing trays.
    ◇ Put together a plate of food, sit down, and interact with others while eating.
    ◇ Eat slowly. This may help you feel full and stop you from going for seconds.

11. Go easy on sweets and high fat desserts:
    ◇ Practice moderation by controlling portion sizes.
    ◇ Share your favorite dessert with a friend.
    ◇ Use Carbohydrate/Fat Exchange List to ensure balance.

12. Stay active:
    ◇ Move more and move faster.
    ◇ Count your daily steps and meet your daily goals.
    ◇ Use stairs when you can.
    ◇ Walk before and, if possible, after your holiday meal.

13. Lastly, think of some family or solitary activities that bring you joy.

The Path to Success

Diet:
- » 3 well-balanced meals
- » Healthy snacks in between B, L, D
- » Limit processed foods
- » Eat out fewer than 3 times per week
- » Limit drinking
- » _____
- » _____

Activity:
- » Total of 45 to 60 minutes of daily aerobic activities (i.e., Brisk walking)
- » Weight bearing exercises three times per week (Low intensity)
- » Limit sedentary activities
- » _____
- » _____

Behavior:
- » Make reasonable and realistic plans
- » Use the STOP Sign
- » Weigh weekly
- » Keep daily food logs (refer to 21-Day Log Book for Achieving Wellness Goals)
- » Count calories
- » Set limits
- » Change your mindset (i.e., see regressions and relapses to old patterns as an opportunity for growth and change)
- » Learn from setbacks through Genuine Accountability Process (refer to Accountability and Empowerment)
- » Be true to yourself
- » _____
- » _____

YOUR DAILY DIET GOAL

FOOD GROUPS	NUMBER OF SERVINGS				
	Breakfast	Snack	Lunch	Snack	Dinner
Grains 1 Serving = 80 Calories					
Starchy Vegetables and Legumes 1 Serving = 80 Calories					
Vegetables: Raw and Cooked 1 Serving = 25 Calories *(1 cup raw or 1/2 cup cooked)*					
Fruits 1 Serving = 60 Calories					
Dairy (1 Serving = 90-120 Calories)					
Meats and Meat substitutes (1 Serving = Varies)					
Fats (1 Serving = 45 Calories)					

Source: 21-Day Log Book for Achieving Wellness Goals

References

Courtney, Mary (2009). *MOSBY'S POCKET GUIDE TO NUTRITIONAL ASSESSMENT AND CARE.* St. Louis, Missouri: Mosby Elsevier.

Escott-Stump, Sylvia, (2015). *NUTRITION AND DIAGNOSIS RELATED CARE* - Eighth Edition. Philadelphia, PA: Wollters Kluwer.

Gilbert, Joyce A. & Schlenker, Eleanor (2019). *WILLIAM'S ESSENTIALS OF NUTRITION AND DIET THERAPY* - Twelfth Edition. St. Louis, Missouri: Mosby Elsevier.

Gropper, Sareen, S., & Smith, Jack, L. (2017). ADVANCED NUTRITION AND HUMAN METABOLISM - Seventh Edition. Boston, MA: Cengage Learning.

Mahan, Kathleen & Raymond, Janice (2016). *KRAUSE'S FOOD & THE NUTRITION CARE PROCESS* - Fourteenth Edition. Philadelphia, PA: Saunders.

Mcintosh, Stacy, N. (2016). *WILLIAM'S BASIC NUTRITION & DIET THERAPY* - Fifteenth Edition. St. Louis, Missouri: Mosby Elsevier.

Nelms, Marcia (2016). *MEDICAL NUTRITION THERAPY: A CASE -STUDY APPROACH.* Boston, MA: Cengage Learning.

Nelms, Marcia & Sucher, Kathryn, P. (2019). *NUTRITION THERAPY AND PATHOPHYSIOLOGY BOOK ONLY* - Fourth Edition. Boston, MA: Cengage Learning.

Noland, Diana, Drisko, Jeanne, A., & Wagner, Leigh (2020). *INTEGRATIVE AND FUNCTIONAL MEDICAL NUTRITION THERAPY*. Totowa, NJ: Humana.

Width, Mary & Reinhard, Tonia (2020). *THE ESSENTIAL POCKET GUIDE FOR CLINICAL NUTRITION* - Third Edition. Burlington, MA: Jones & Bartlett Learning.